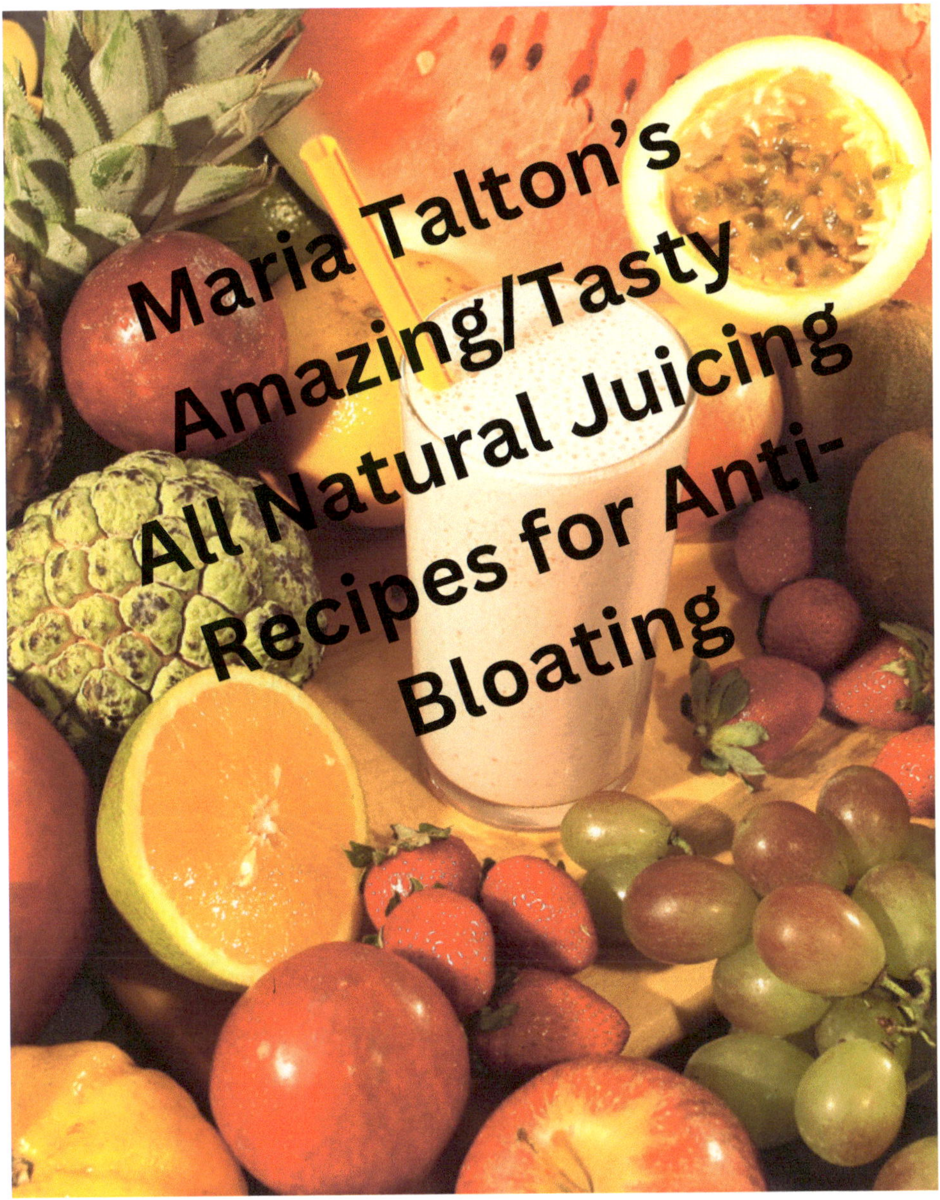

Maria Talton's Amazing/Tasty All Natural Juicing Recipes for Anti-Bloating

INDEX OF RECIPES

JUICES

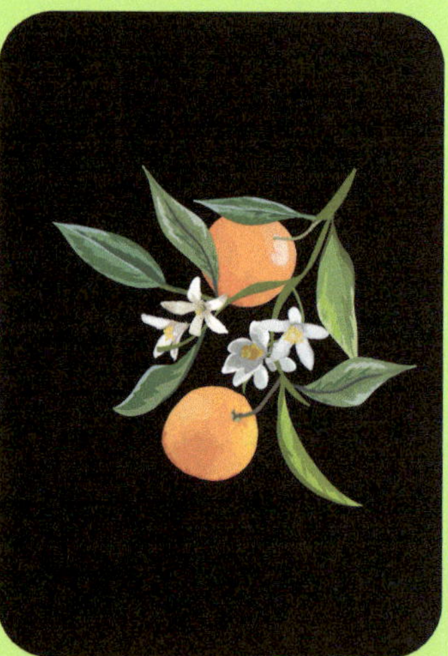

INGREDIENT LIST

- Aloe vera: 3
- Apple cider vinegar: 1
- Beets: 3
- Blueberries: 4
- Carrots: 7
- Celery: 2
- Cilantro: 1
- Coconut water: 1
- Cranberries: 1
- Cucumber: 6
- Fennel: 1
- Ginger: 6
- Green apples: 3
- Green tea: 2
- Kiwi: 4
- Lemon: 9
- Lime: 4
- Mango: 3
- Mint: 11
- Orange: 6
- Papaya: 2
- Parsley: 1
- Peppermint: 1
- Pineapple: 4
- Raspberries: 3
- Spinach: 5
- Strawberries: 5
- Turmeric: 5
- Watermelon: 2

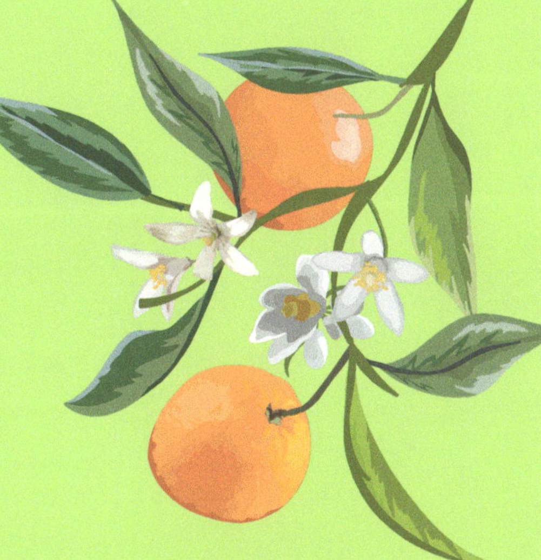

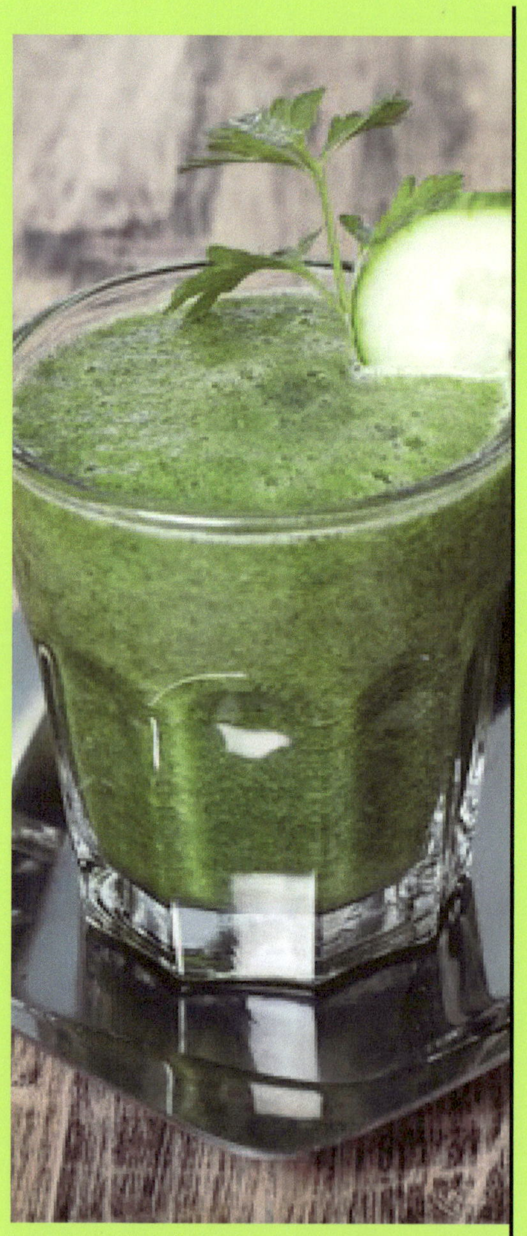

CUCUMBER MINT REFRESHER

Cucumber
Mint
Lemon

Cucumber reduces water retention, mint aids digestion, and lemon supports detoxification, relieving bloating.

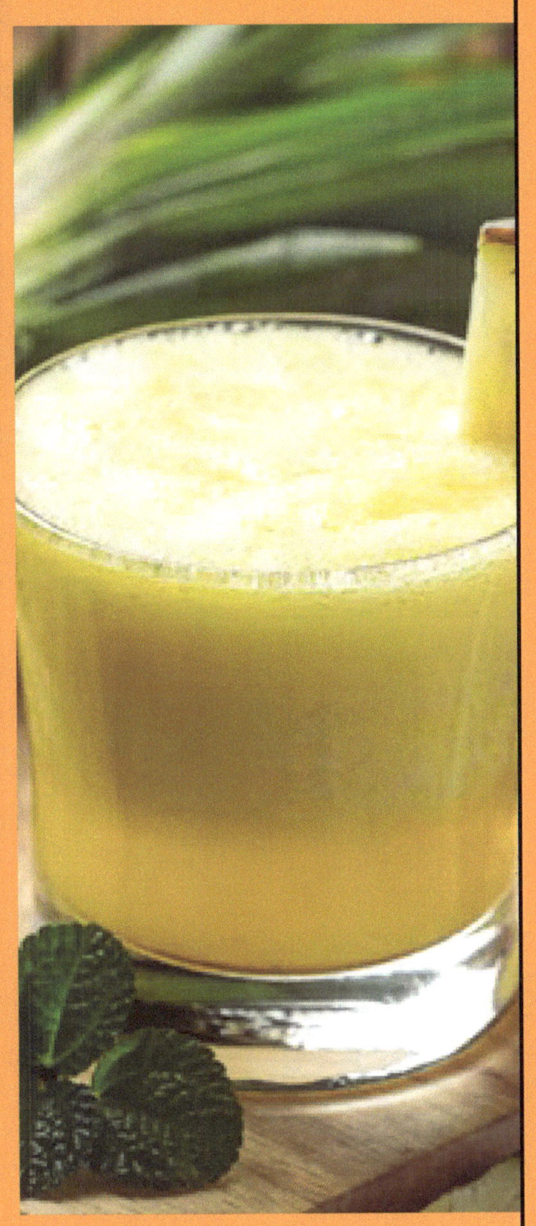

SOOTHING PINEAPPLE GINGER MOCKTAIL

Pineapple
Ginger
Mint
Cucumber

Pineapple contains bromelain, aiding digestion and reducing bloating. Ginger supports digestion and eases bloating.

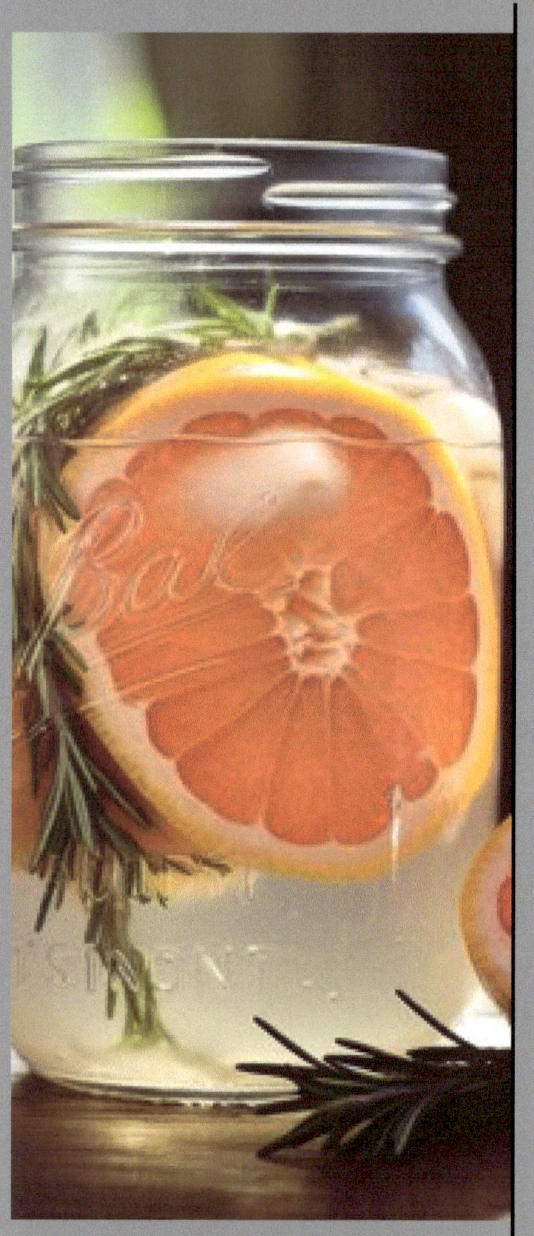

FENNEL CITRUS BEVERAGE

Fennel
Oranges
Mint
Ginger

Fennel relaxes the gastrointestinal tract, oranges provide vitamin C, and mint aids digestion, reducing bloating.

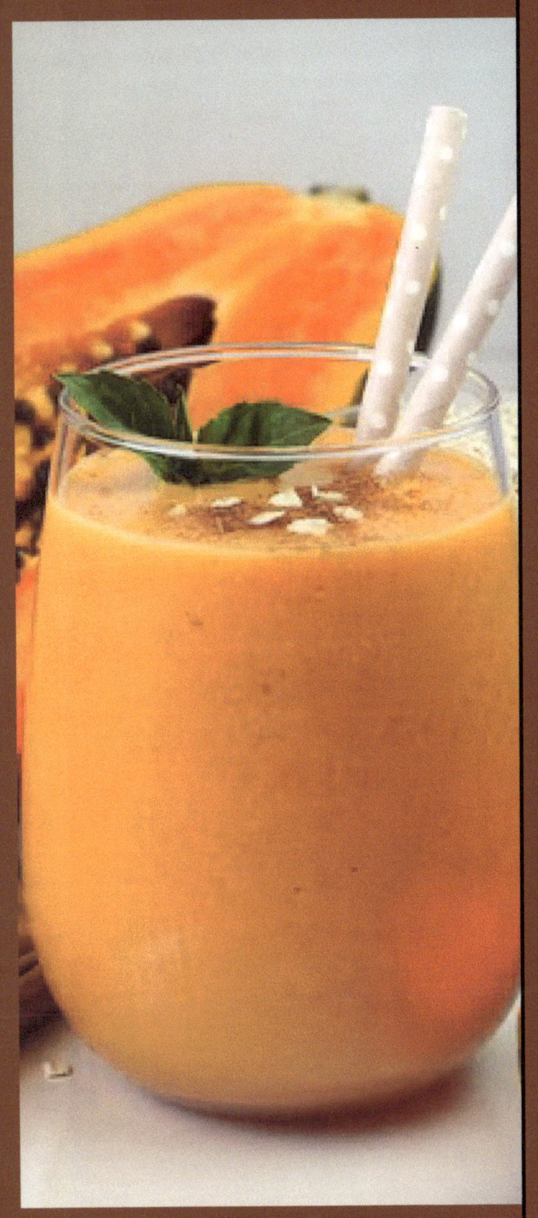

DELIGHTFUL PAPAYA DIGESTIVE DRINK

Papaya
Mint
Lime

Papaya contains enzymes aiding digestion, while mint and lime soothe the digestive system, reducing bloating.

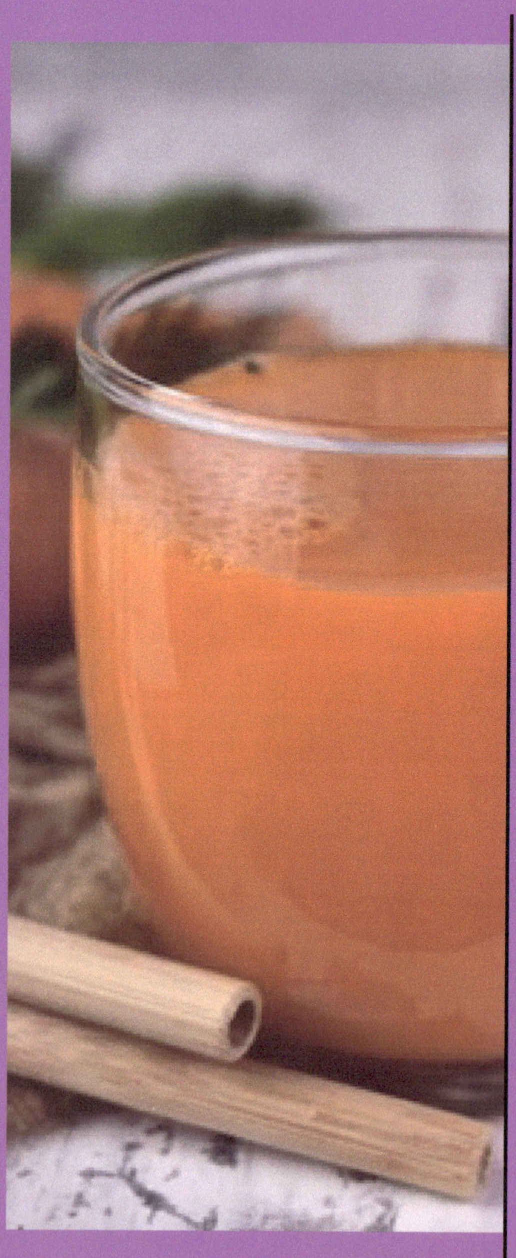

CARROT GINGER DIGESTIVE AID DELICIOUS BEVERAGE

Carrots
Ginger
Turmeric
Lemon

Carrots are gentle on the digestive system, ginger aids digestion, turmeric reduces inflammation, reducing bloating.

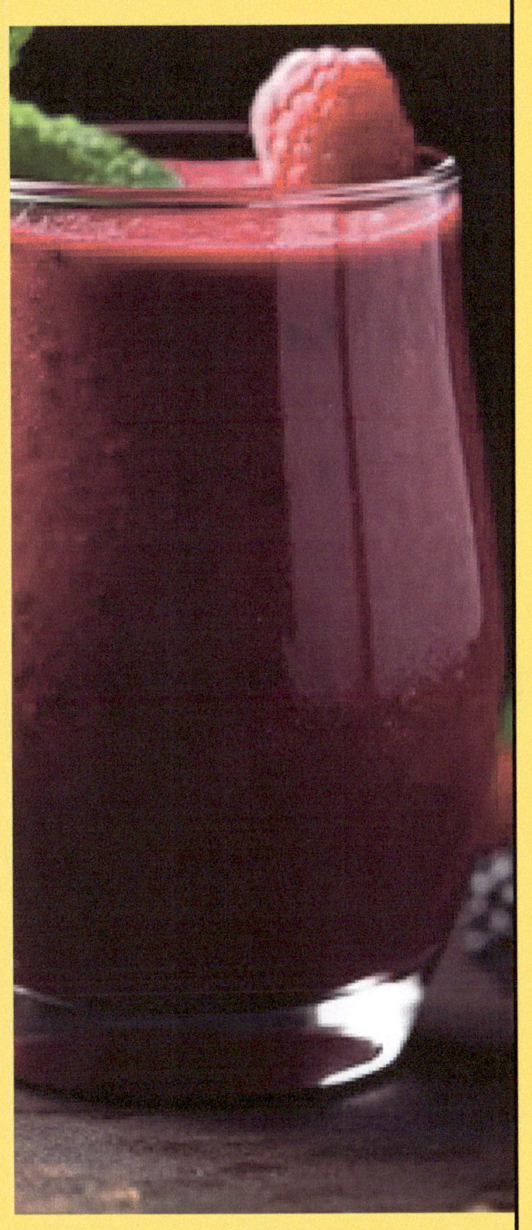

SMASHING BERRY BLOAT BUSTER

Blueberries
Raspberries
Strawberries
Mint

Berries are rich in fiber, aiding digestion, while mint soothes the digestive tract, reducing bloating.

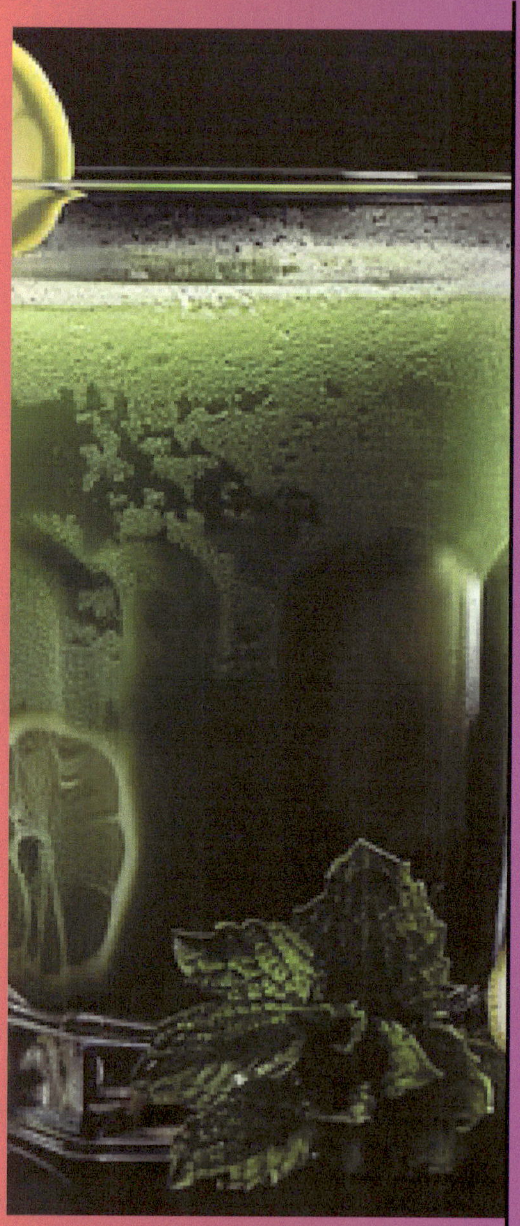

CILANTRO LEMON DETOX REFRESHER

Cilantro
Lemon
Cucumber

Cilantro supports digestion and detoxification, lemon aids digestion, and cucumber reduces water retention and bloating.

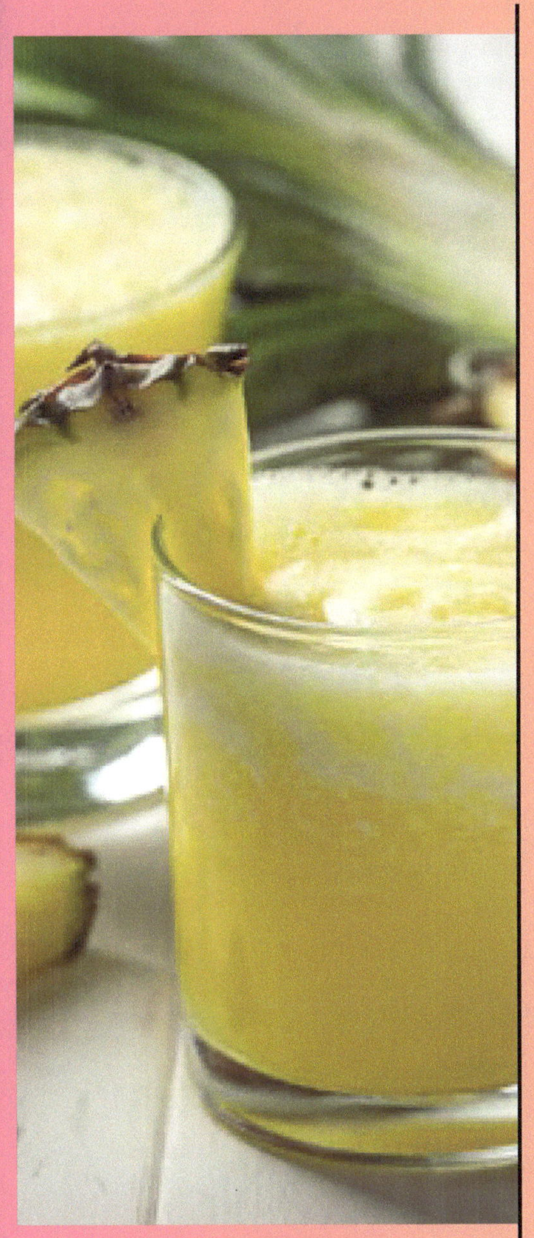

PINEAPPLE CUCUMBER HYDRATING JUICE

Pineapple
Cucumber
Aloe vera
Mint

Pineapple aids digestion, cucumber reduces water retention, aloe vera soothes the digestive tract, reducing bloating.

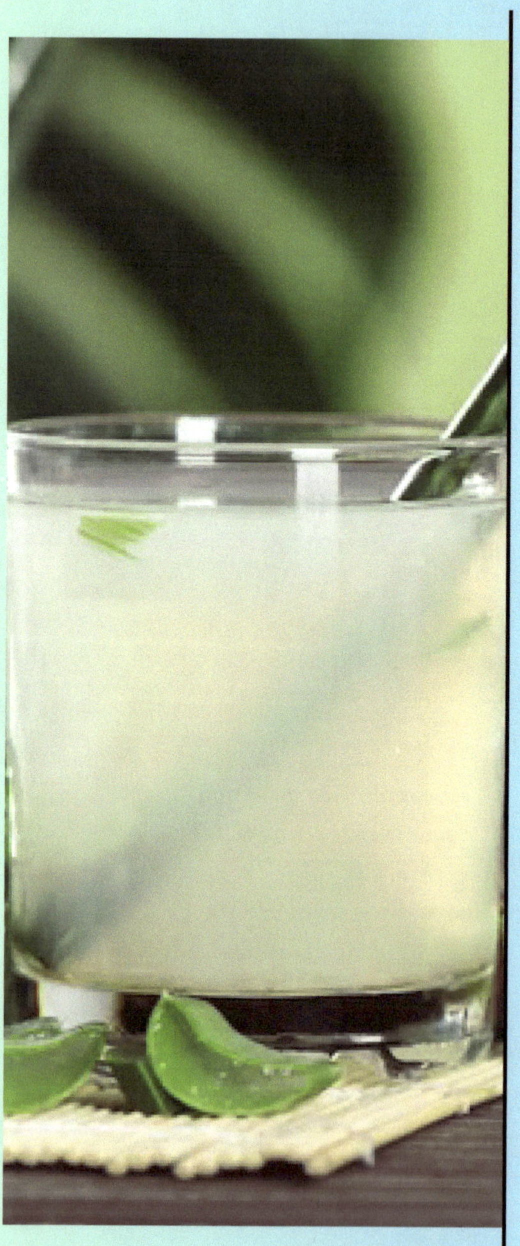

LEMON ALOE VERA DIGESTIVE TONIC

Lemon
Aloe vera
Mint

Lemon supports digestion, aloe vera soothes the digestive tract, and mint aids in reducing bloating and discomfort.

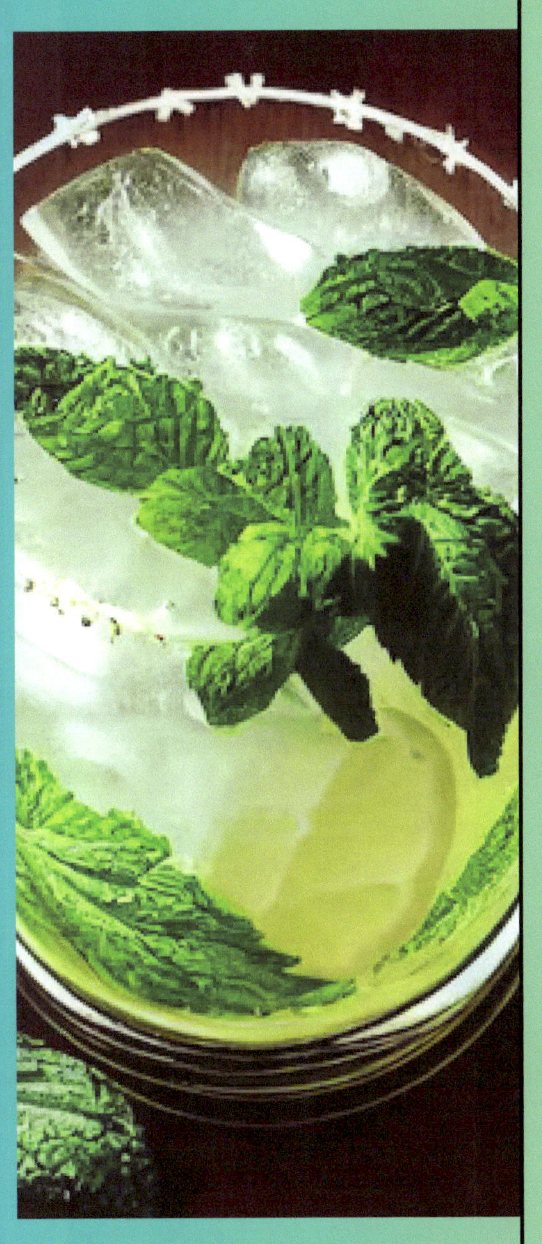

GREEN TEA PEPPERMINT REJUVENATOR

Green tea
Peppermint
Lemon

Green tea aids digestion, peppermint relaxes the digestive tract, and lemon adds a burst of vitamin C, reducing bloating.

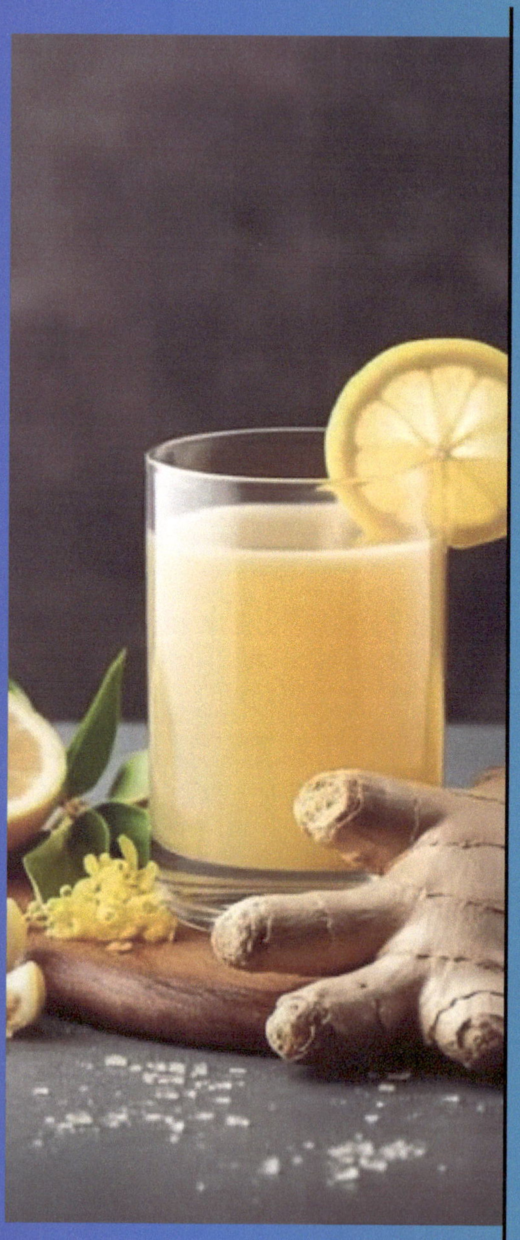

GINGER TURMERIC DIGESTIVE DELIGHT

Ginger
Turmeric
Pineapple
Lemon

Ginger and turmeric are anti-inflammatory, aiding digestion and reducing bloating, while pineapple adds a tropical flavor.

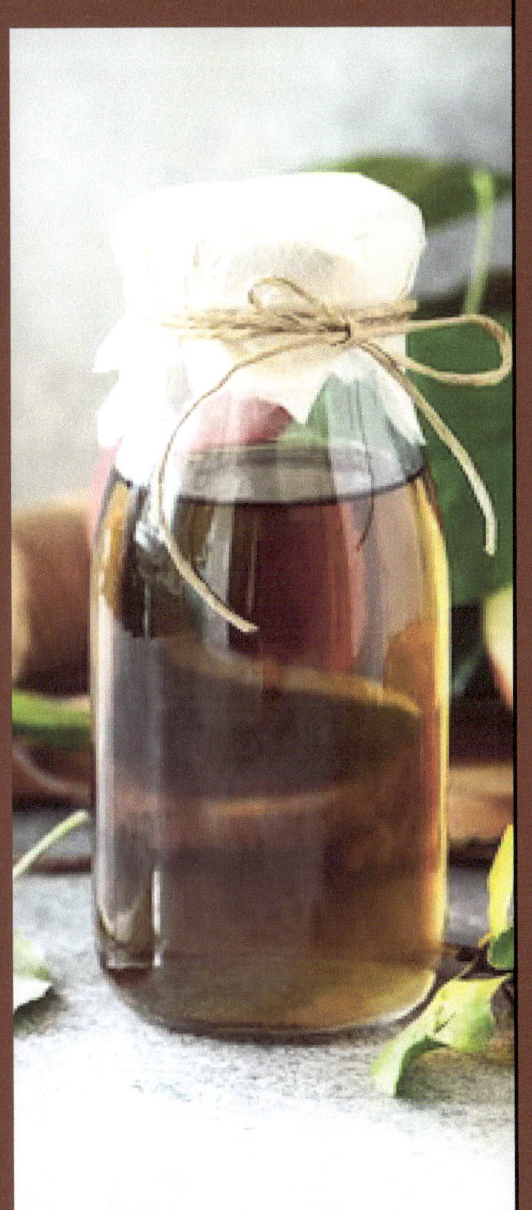

APPLE CIDER VINEGAR DIGESTIVE ELIXIR

Apple cider vinegar
Green apples
Lemon

Apple cider vinegar
supports digestion and may
reduce bloating, and green
apples provide fiber and
aid in digestion.

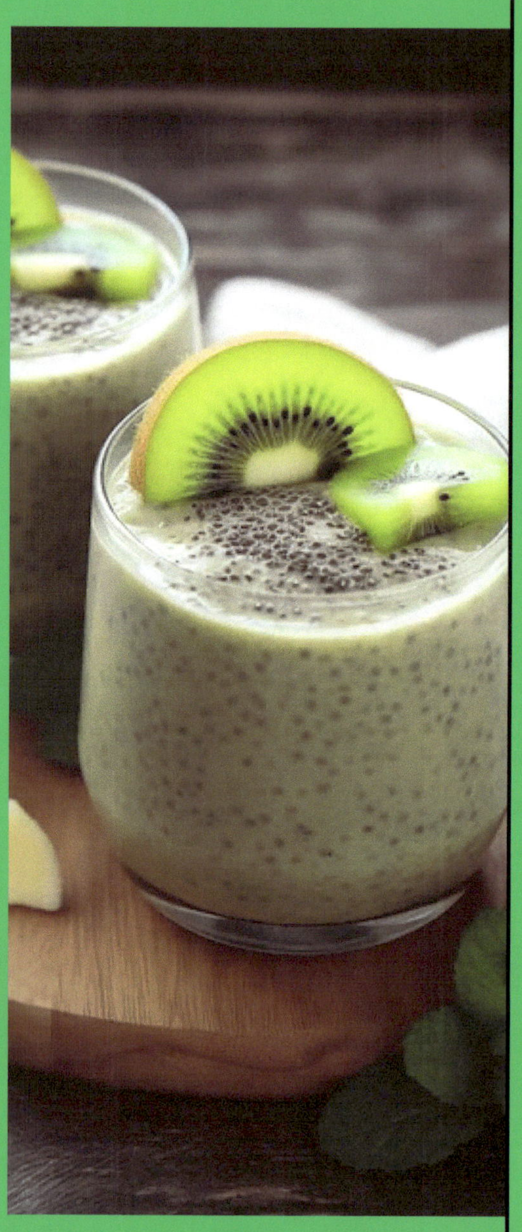

KIWI PAPAYA DIGESTIVE SOUTHERN SMOOTHIE

Kiwi
Papaya
Mint
Coconut water

Kiwi and papaya aid digestion, while mint soothes the digestive tract, and coconut water helps with hydration and bloating.

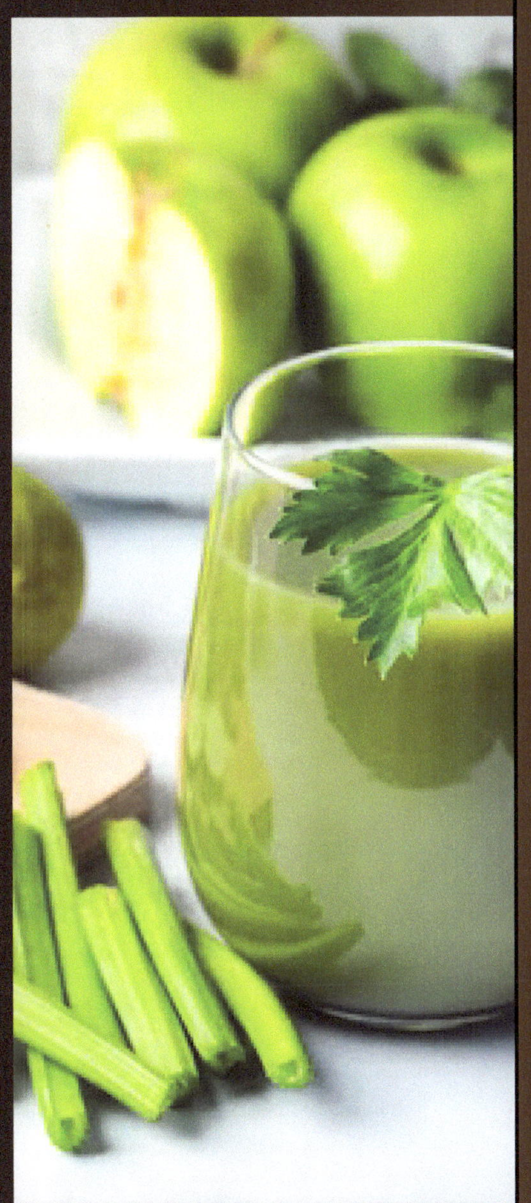

SPINACH CUCUMBER CELERY DIGESTION CLEANSER

Spinach
Cucumber
Celery
Lemon

Spinach is hydrating and aids digestion, cucumber reduces water retention, celery supports digestion, reducing bloating.

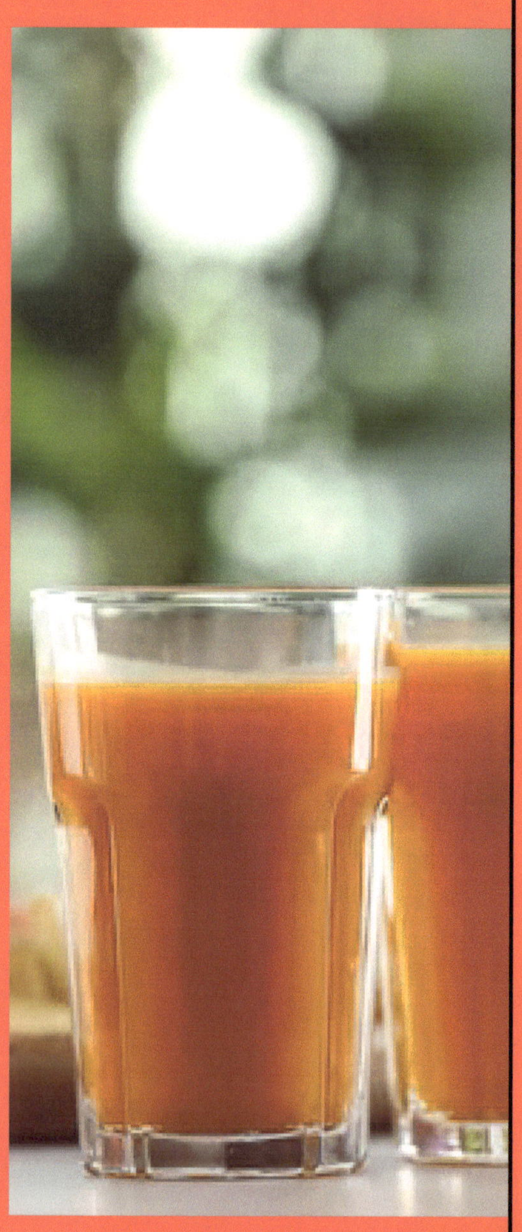

TURMERIC CARROT DIGESTIVE HELPER

Turmeric
Carrots
Oranges
Ginger

Turmeric and ginger are anti-inflammatory, aiding digestion and reducing bloating, while carrots and oranges provide essential nutrients.

17

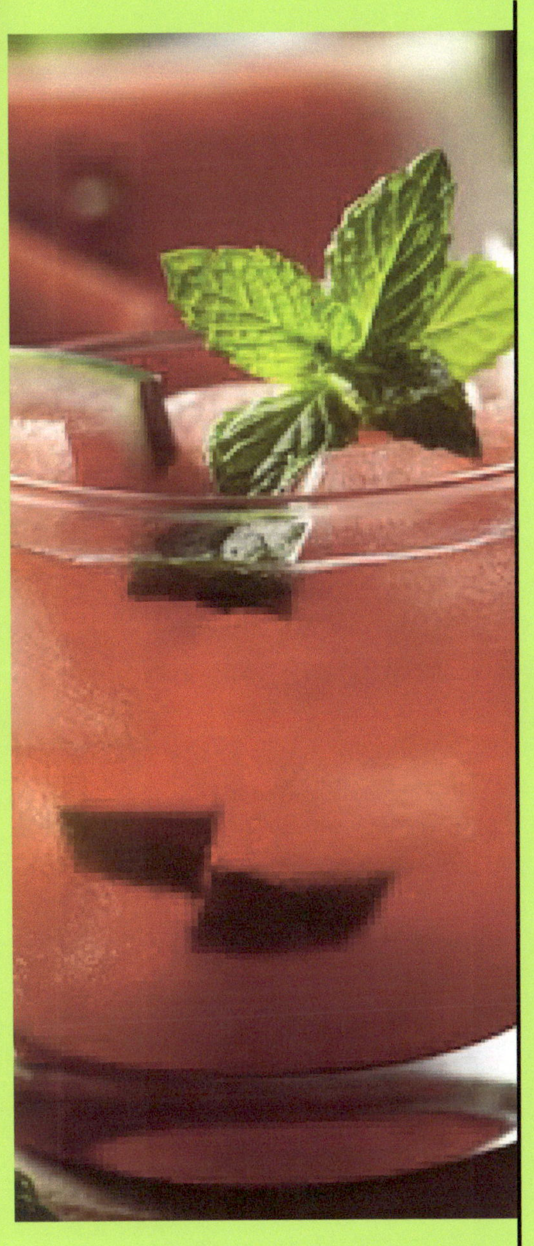

WATERMELON MINT HYDRATION BOOSTER

Watermelon
Mint
Lime

Watermelon is hydrating and may reduce water retention, mint soothes the digestive tract, and lime provides vitamin C.

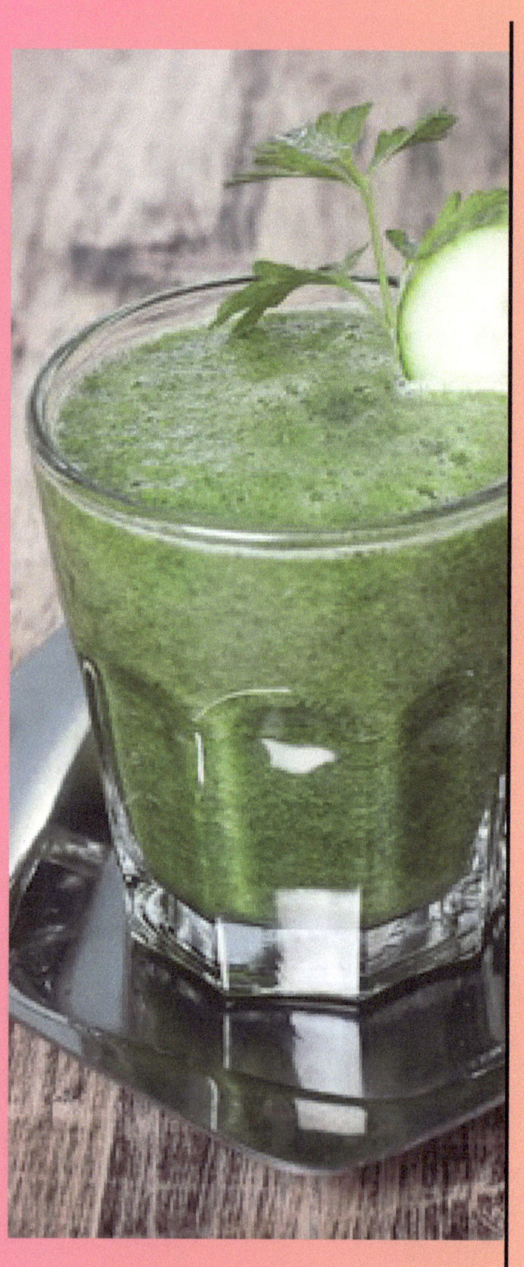

CUCUMBER LEMON PARSLEY HEALTHY COOLER

Cucumber
Lemon
Parsley

Cucumber reduces water retention, lemon aids digestion, and parsley supports overall digestive health, reducing bloating.

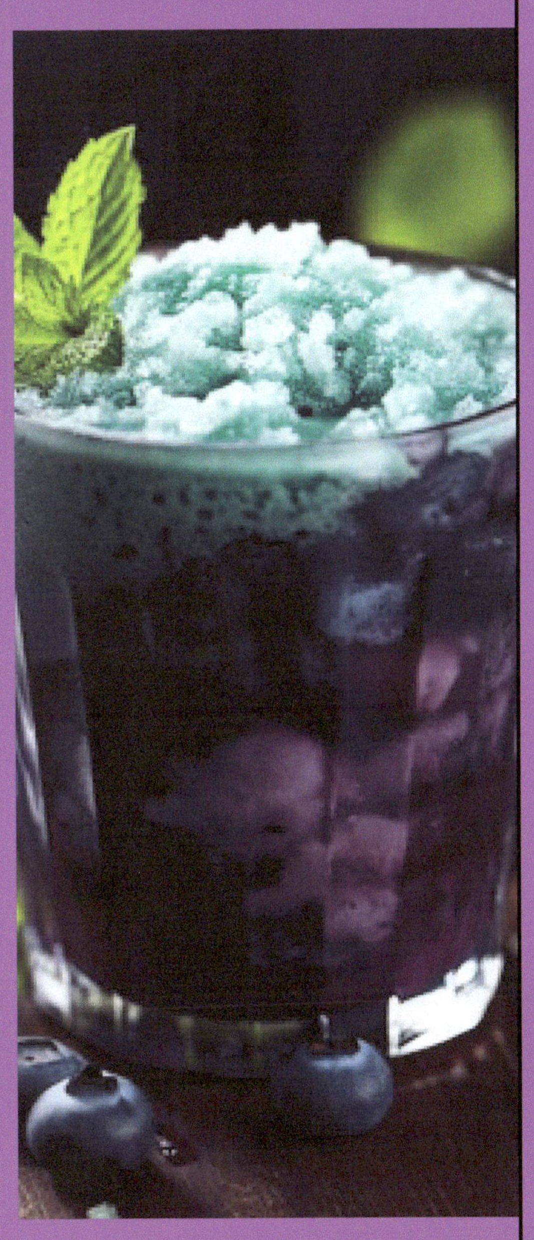

BLUEBERRY MINT DIGESTIVE REFRESHING MOCKTAIL

Blueberries
Mint
Cucumber
Lime

Blueberries aid digestion, mint soothes the digestive tract, cucumber reduces water retention, and lime provides vitamin C.

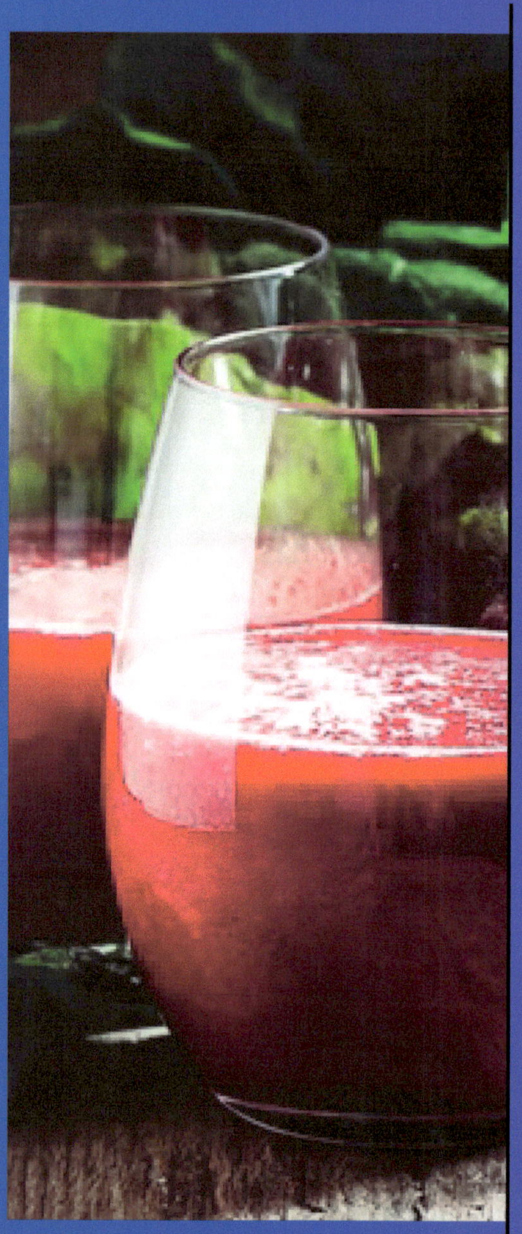

BEETROOT
CARROT DETOX

Beets
Carrots
Lemon

Beets and carrots support liver function and digestion, lemon aids detoxification, and together they reduce bloating.

21

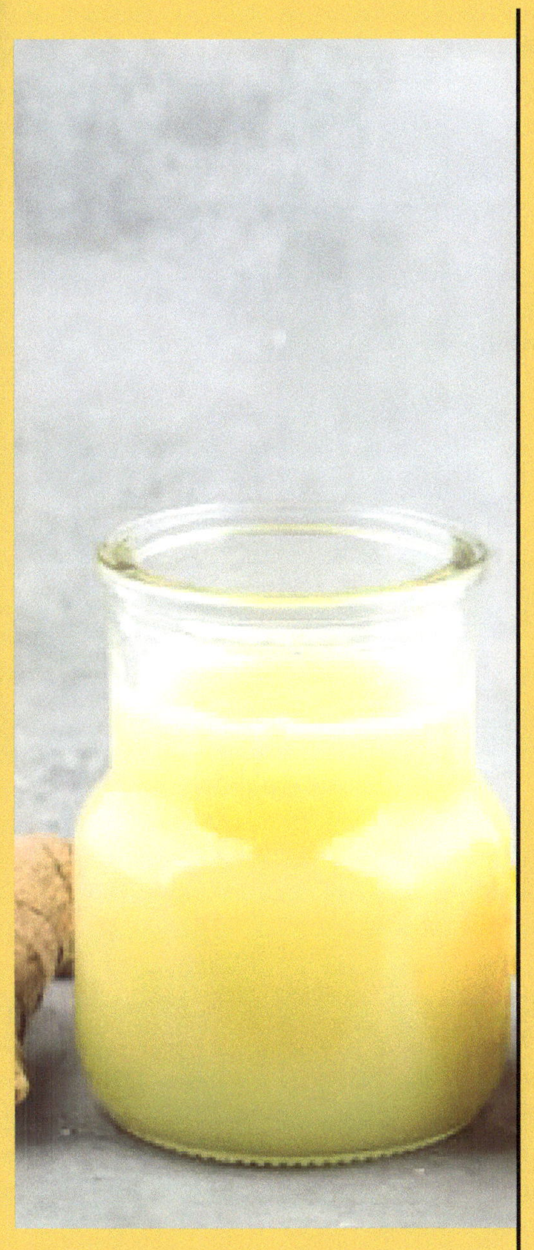

ORANGE GINGER DIGESTIVE CONCOCTION

Oranges
Ginger
Mint

Oranges provide vitamin C and aid digestion, ginger supports digestion and reduces bloating, while mint adds a refreshing taste.

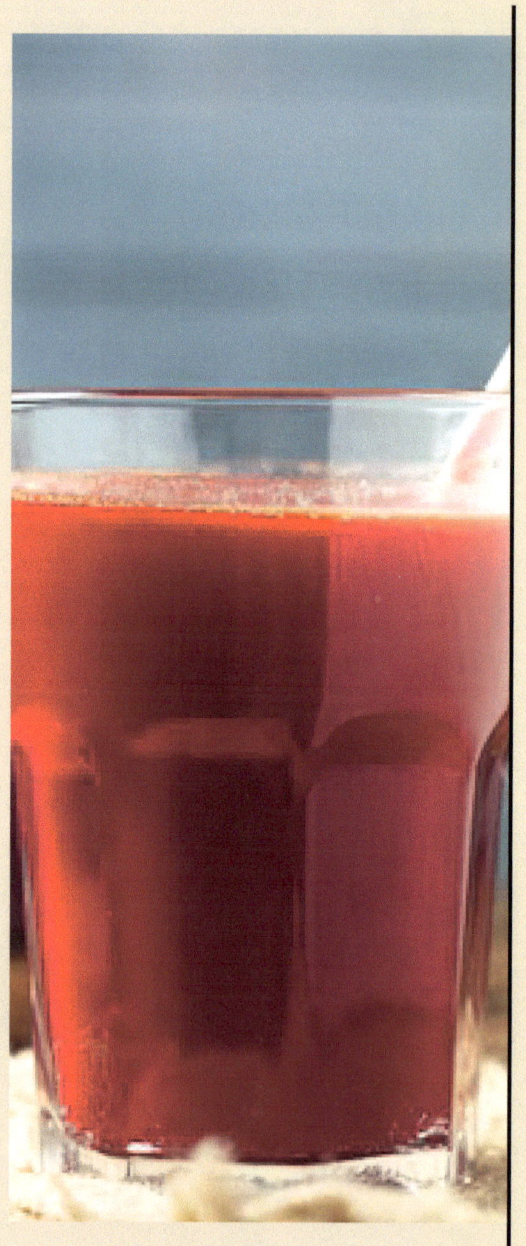

CRANBERRY GINGER DETOX COOLER

Cranberries
Ginger
Cucumbers
Lemon

Cranberries are antioxidant-rich, ginger aids digestion, cucumbers reduce water retention, and lemon aids detoxification.

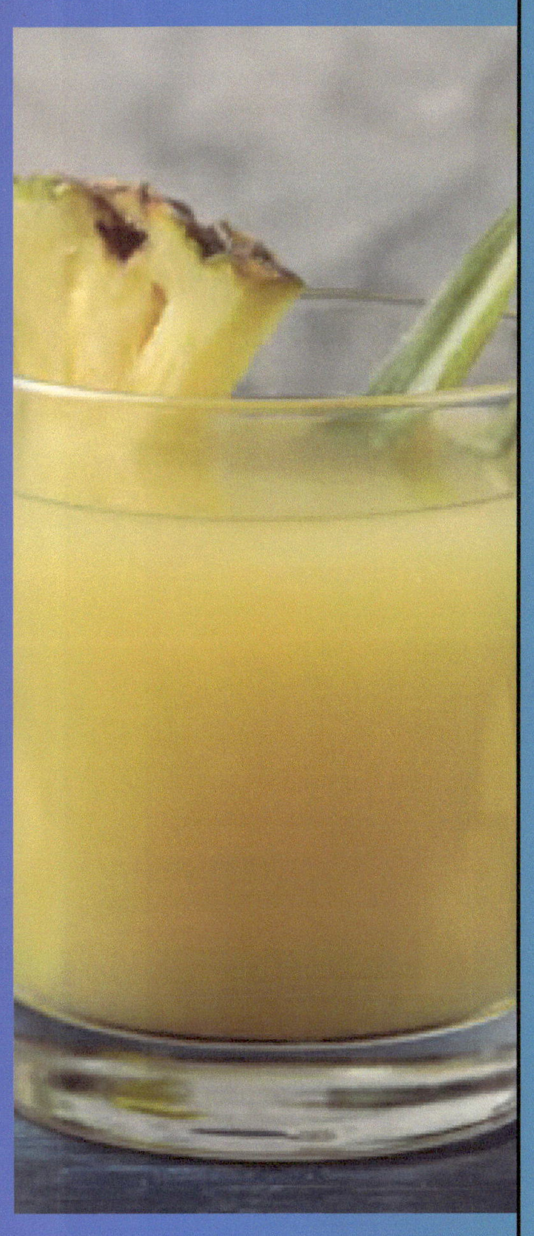

ALOE VERA PINEAPPLE DIGESTIVE JUICE

Aloe vera
Pineapple
Mint

Aloe vera supports digestion and soothes the digestive tract, pineapple aids digestion, and mint adds a refreshing flavor.

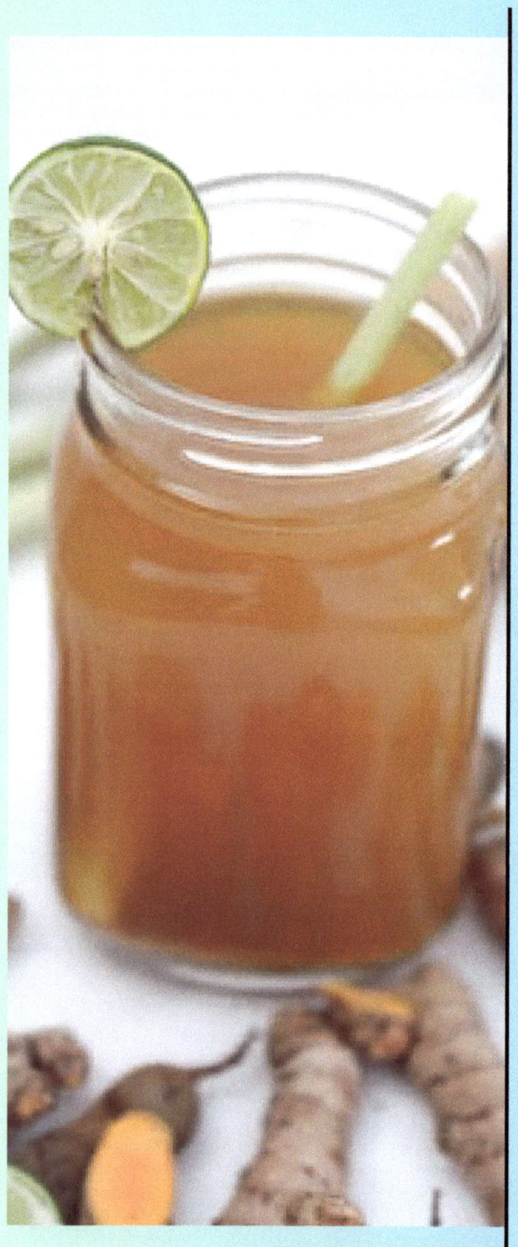

CARROT ORANGE TURMERIC CLEANSER

Carrots
Oranges
Turmeric
Ginger

Carrots and oranges aid digestion, turmeric reduces inflammation, ginger supports digestion, reducing bloating.

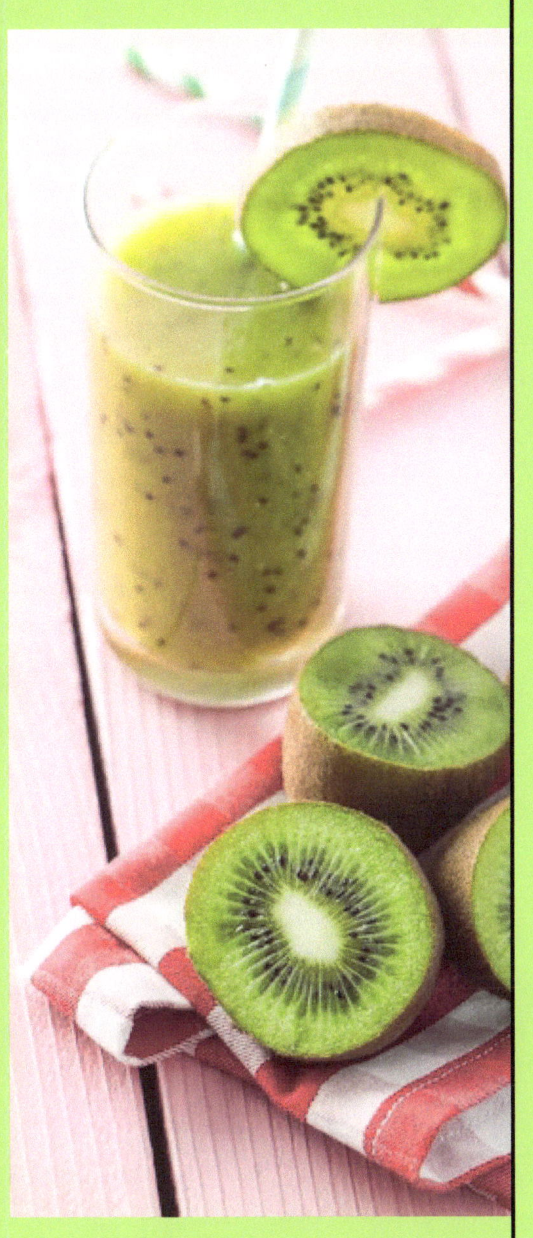

GREEN APPLE KIWI DIGESTIVE SUPERJUICE

Green apples
Kiwi
Lemon
Ginger

Green apples and kiwi aid digestion, lemon supports detoxification, ginger reduces bloating, and aids digestion.

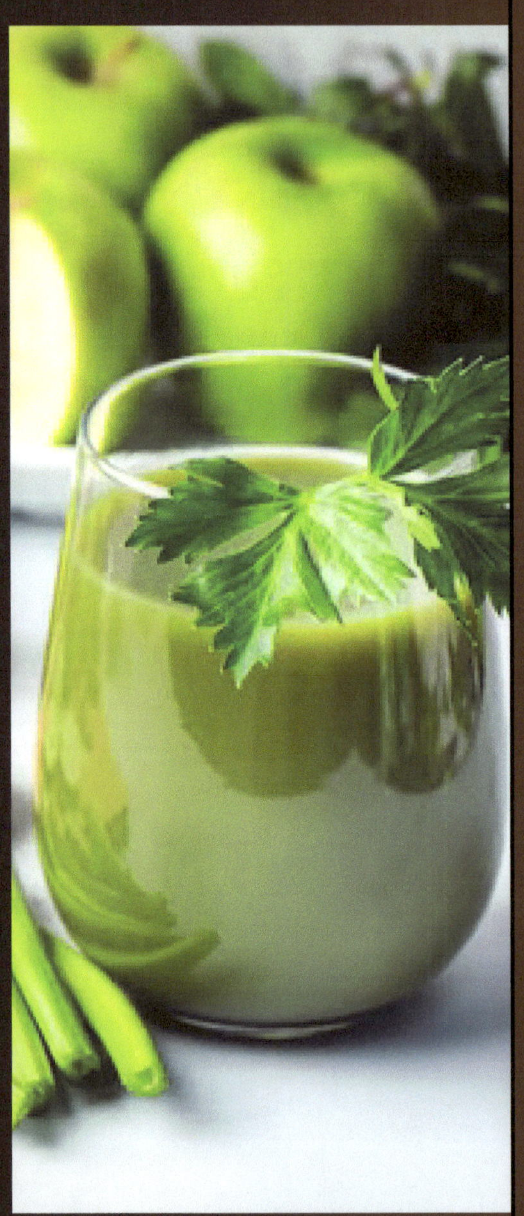

CELERY
CUCUMBER
HYDRATION
POWERHOUSE

Celery
Cucumber
Spinach
Mint

**Celery and cucumber
reduce water retention,
spinach adds nutrients,
mint soothes digestion,
aiding in reducing bloating.**

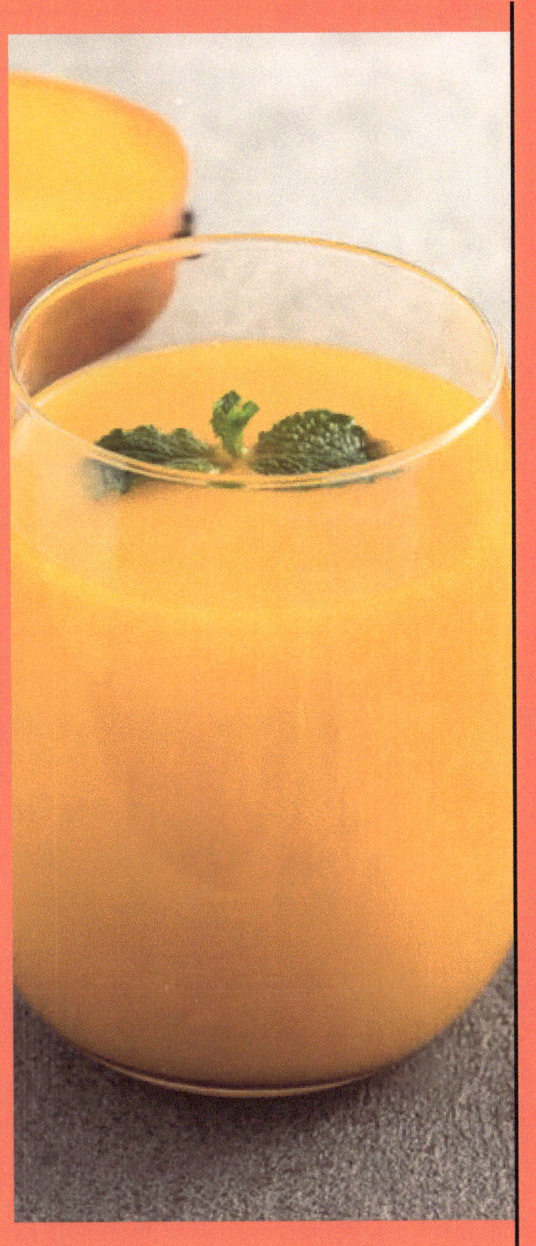

MANGO PAPAYA DIGESTIVE SOOTHING SMOOTHIE

Mango
Papaya
Lime

Mango and papaya aid digestion, lime adds vitamin C, and together they provide a tropical and soothing digestive smoothie.

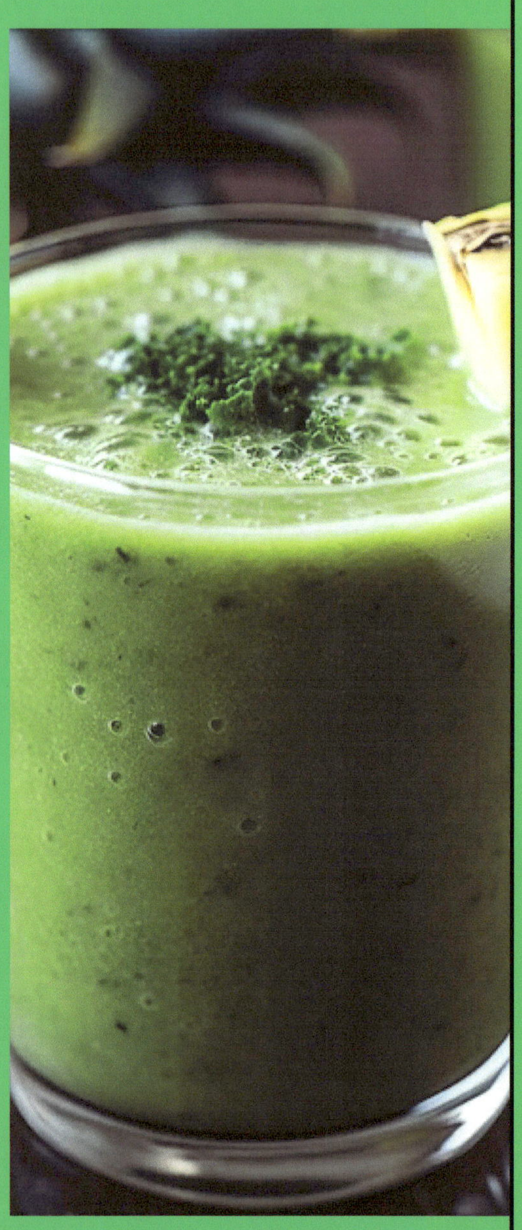

SPINACH
PINEAPPLE
DIGESTIVE ELIXIR

Spinach
Pineapple
Ginger
Lemon

Spinach aids digestion, pineapple provides bromelain for digestion, ginger reduces bloating, and lemon aids detoxification.

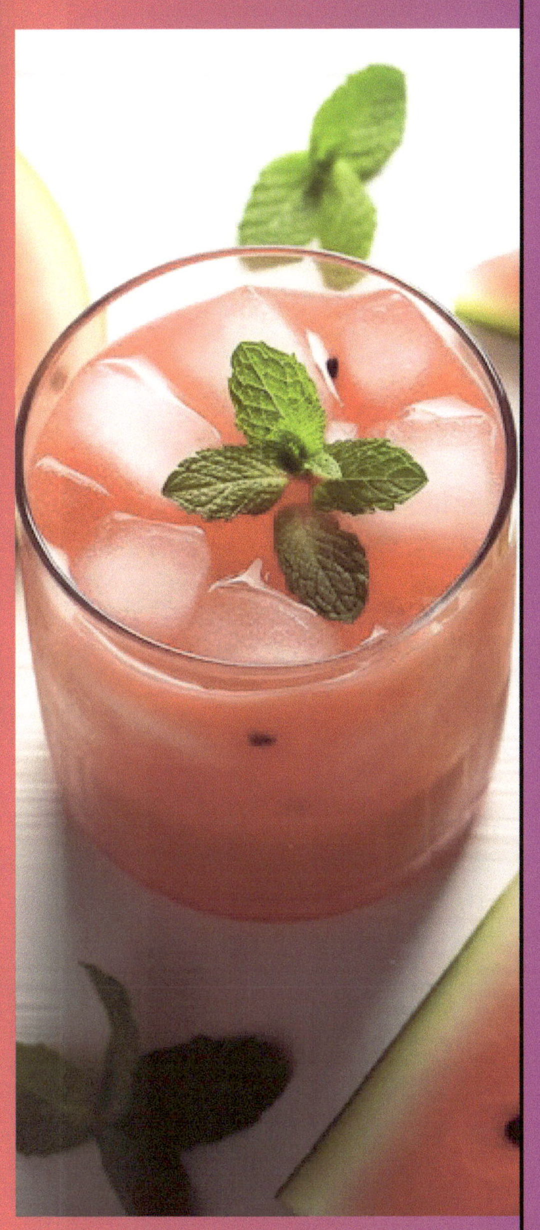

WATERMELON CUCUMBER MINT REFRESHING TREAT

Watermelon
Cucumber
Mint
Lime

Watermelon hydrates and may reduce water retention, cucumber reduces bloating, and mint adds a refreshing flavor.

30

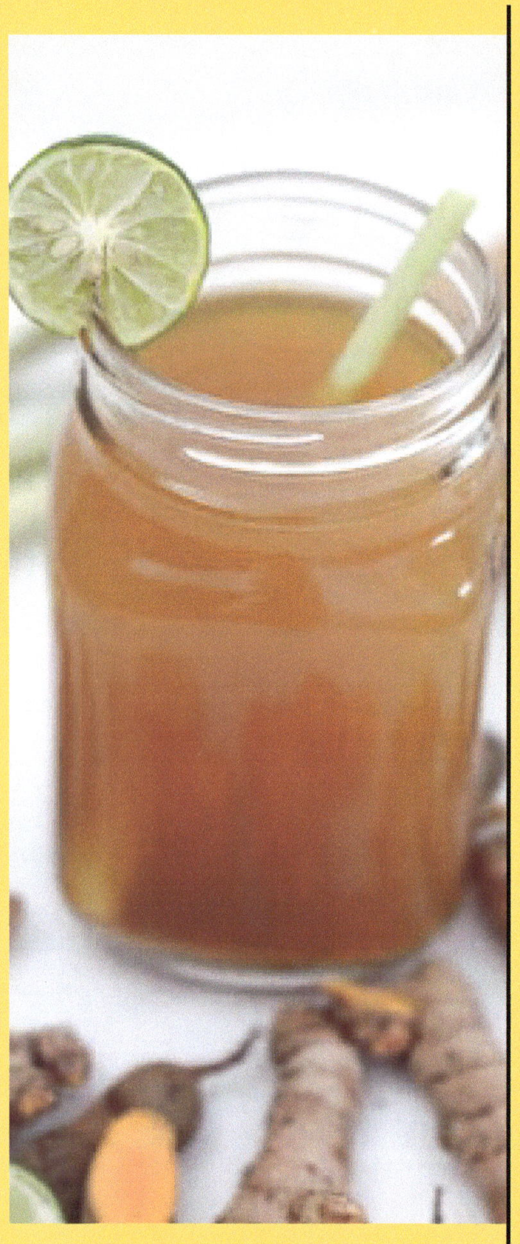

CARROT GINGER MINT ANTI-BLOATING TONIC

Carrots
Ginger
Mint
Lemon

Carrots aid digestion, ginger reduces bloating, mint soothes the digestive tract, and lemon adds a burst of vitamin C.

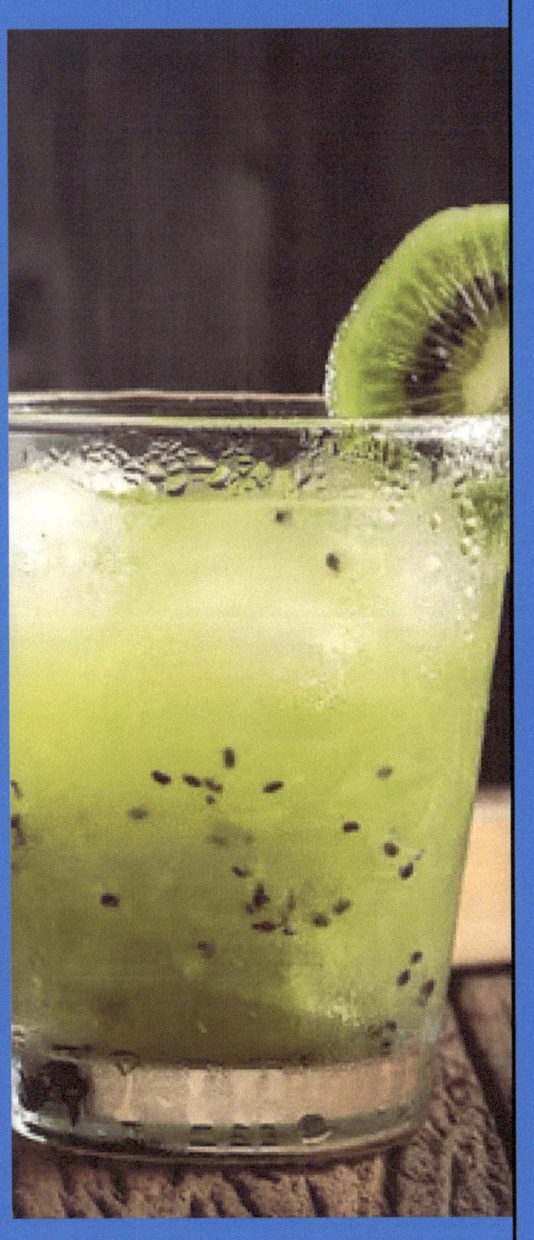

KIWI PINEAPPLE DELICIOUS BLEND

Kiwi
Pineapple
Cucumber
Mint

Kiwi and pineapple aid digestion, cucumber reduces water retention, mint soothes the digestive tract, reducing bloating.

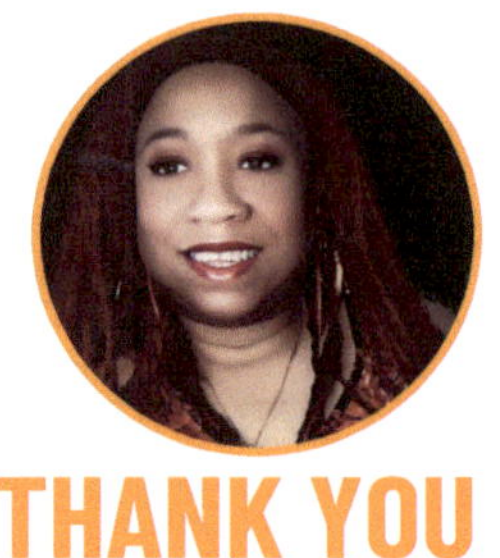

THANK YOU

Unlock the Secrets of Anti-Bloating Juicing: A Guide to Natural Wellness

In the quest for a healthier lifestyle, juicing has emerged as a popular and effective method to boost wellness, detoxify the body, and address common issues such as bloating. My latest book, an anti-bloating juicing guide, is designed to help you on this journey. While it does not provide specific quantities for each ingredient, it serves as a comprehensive guide to show you which fruits and vegetables work synergistically to support your body's natural functions.

Discover the Power of Natural Ingredients

This book is a celebration of the incredible benefits that natural ingredients can offer. Through careful selection of fruits and vegetables, it highlights combinations that not only taste great but also work together to reduce bloating and improve digestion. By understanding the natural properties of each ingredient, you can create juices that are both delicious and beneficial for your body.

Embrace Creativity in Your Juicing Journey

One of the unique aspects of this book is its focus on encouraging creativity in your juicing process. Instead of providing rigid recipes with exact measurements, it empowers you to experiment with different combinations and quantities. This approach allows you to tailor your juices to your personal taste preferences and nutritional needs, making the process both enjoyable and customizable.

Key Combinations for Anti-Bloating

This book showcases a variety of fruits and vegetables known for their anti-bloating properties. For instance:
- **Cucumber and Mint**: These ingredients are refreshing and help to reduce water retention.
- **Pineapple and Ginger**: Pineapple contains bromelain, an enzyme that aids digestion, while ginger soothes the digestive tract.
- **Apple and Fennel**: Apples provide fiber, and fennel has natural diuretic properties.

By understanding these combinations, you can create juices that target bloating and promote a flatter, more comfortable abdomen.

The Natural Collective: Synergy of Ingredients

The concept of a natural collective is central to this book. It emphasizes how different ingredients can work together to enhance each other's benefits. For example, pairing hydrating fruits like watermelon with anti-inflammatory herbs like basil creates a powerful blend that supports overall digestive health.

A Creative Endeavor

This book is more than just a guide; it is a creative endeavor meant to inspire and support your journey toward natural wellness. We hope that by exploring the combinations and experimenting with your own recipes, you will discover the joy and benefits of juicing.

Thank you for being a part of this creative journey. I am excited to see how these ideas will help you move forward on your path to health and wellness through natural juicing. Enjoy the process, and happy juicing!

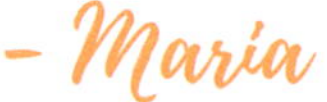